Dedication

To all my little ones who love their fruits. I know that you will enjoy this book. It was made for you.

FRUITS OOOH FRUITS

WRITTEN AND ILLUSTRATED
BY DENISE BRACKETT

Fruits are good for us in so many ways. God made many different types of fruits, too many to tell here. Let's take a look at a few of the ones that can be found in our markets and supermarkets, and some of the ways they help our bodies.

LET'S GO...

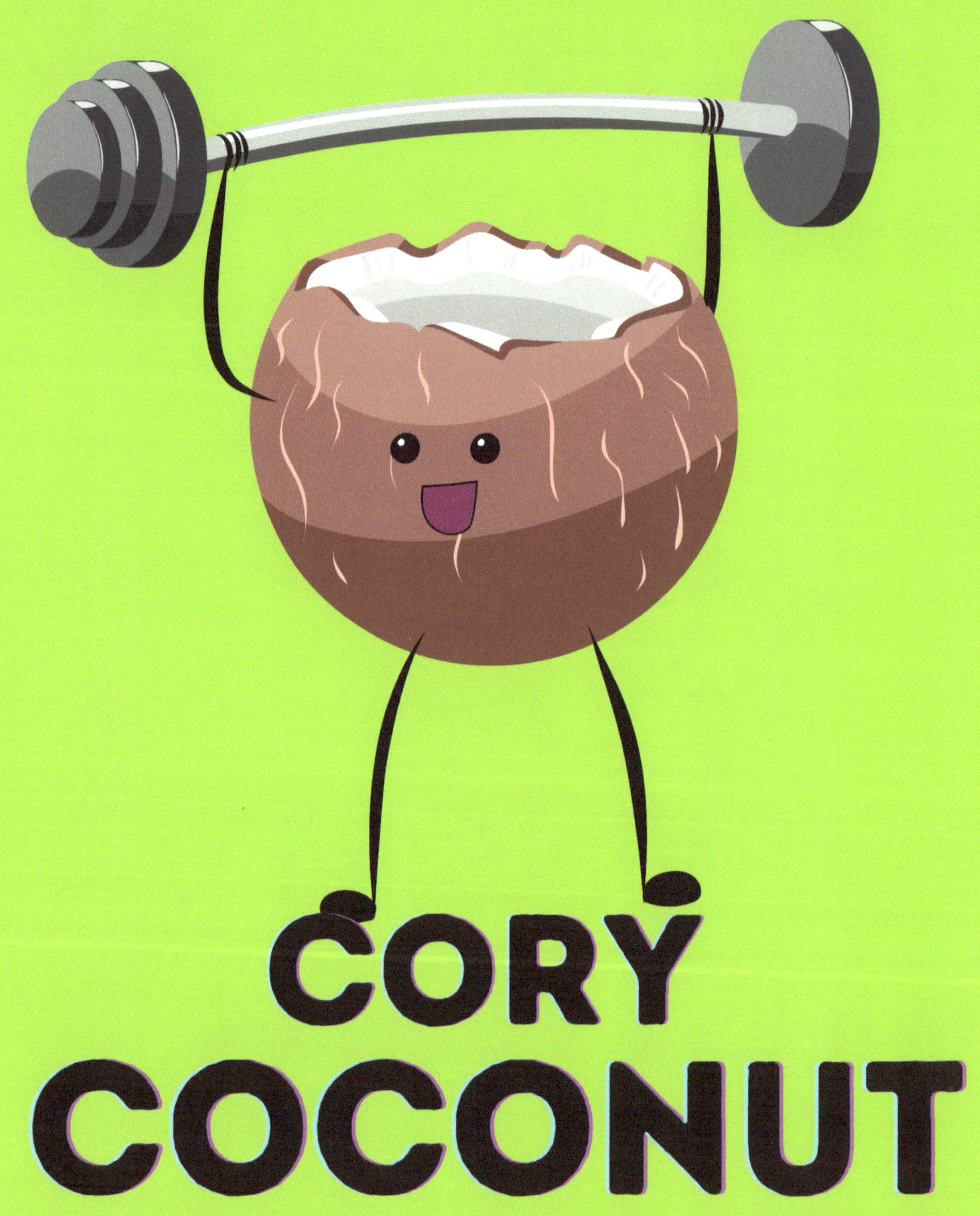

CORY
COCONUT

COCONUTS ARE GOOD FOR YOUR TEETH AND BONES.

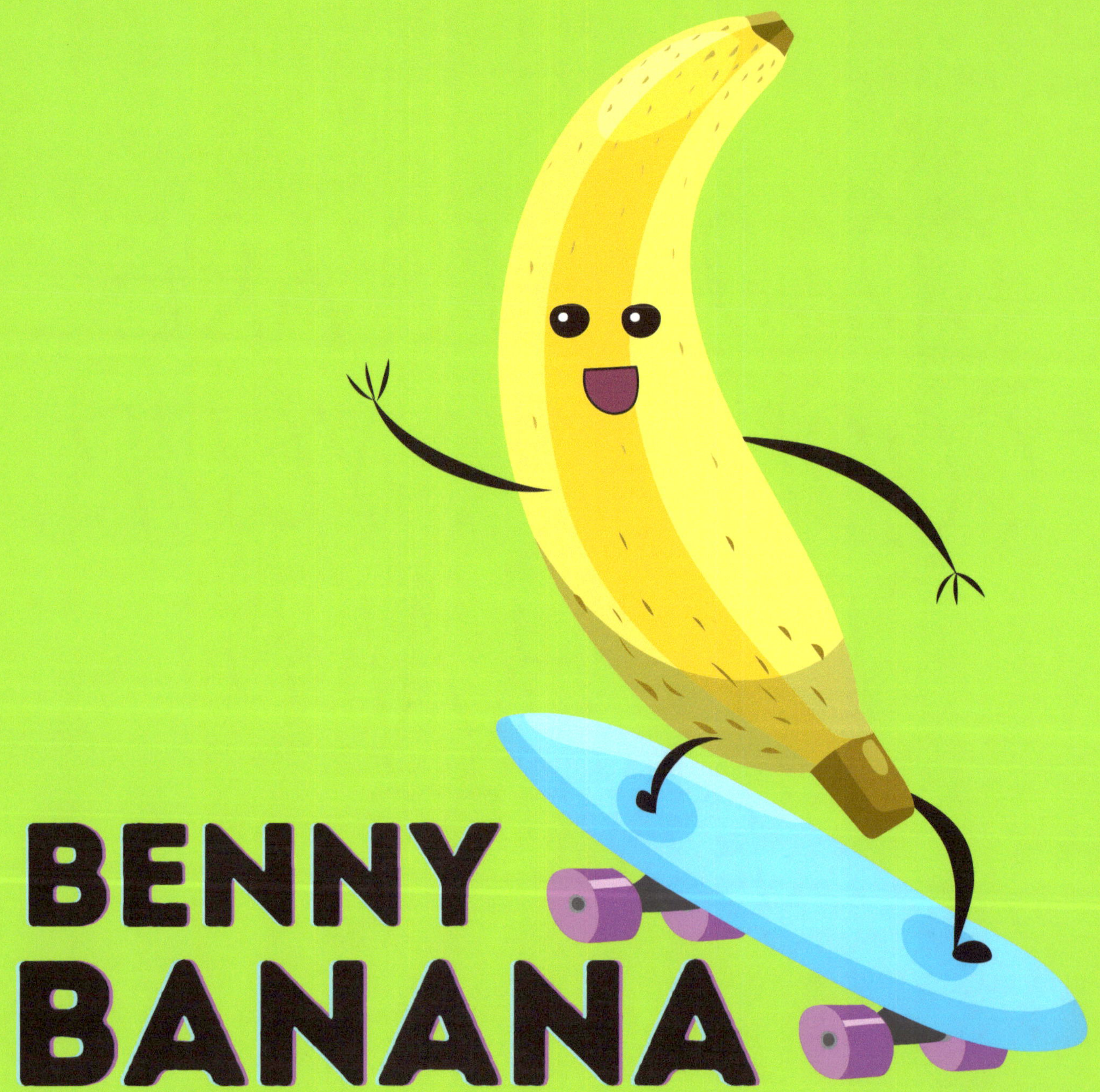

BENNY
BANANA

BANANAS GIVE
YOU ENERGY
AND ARE GOOD
FOR YOUR BONES

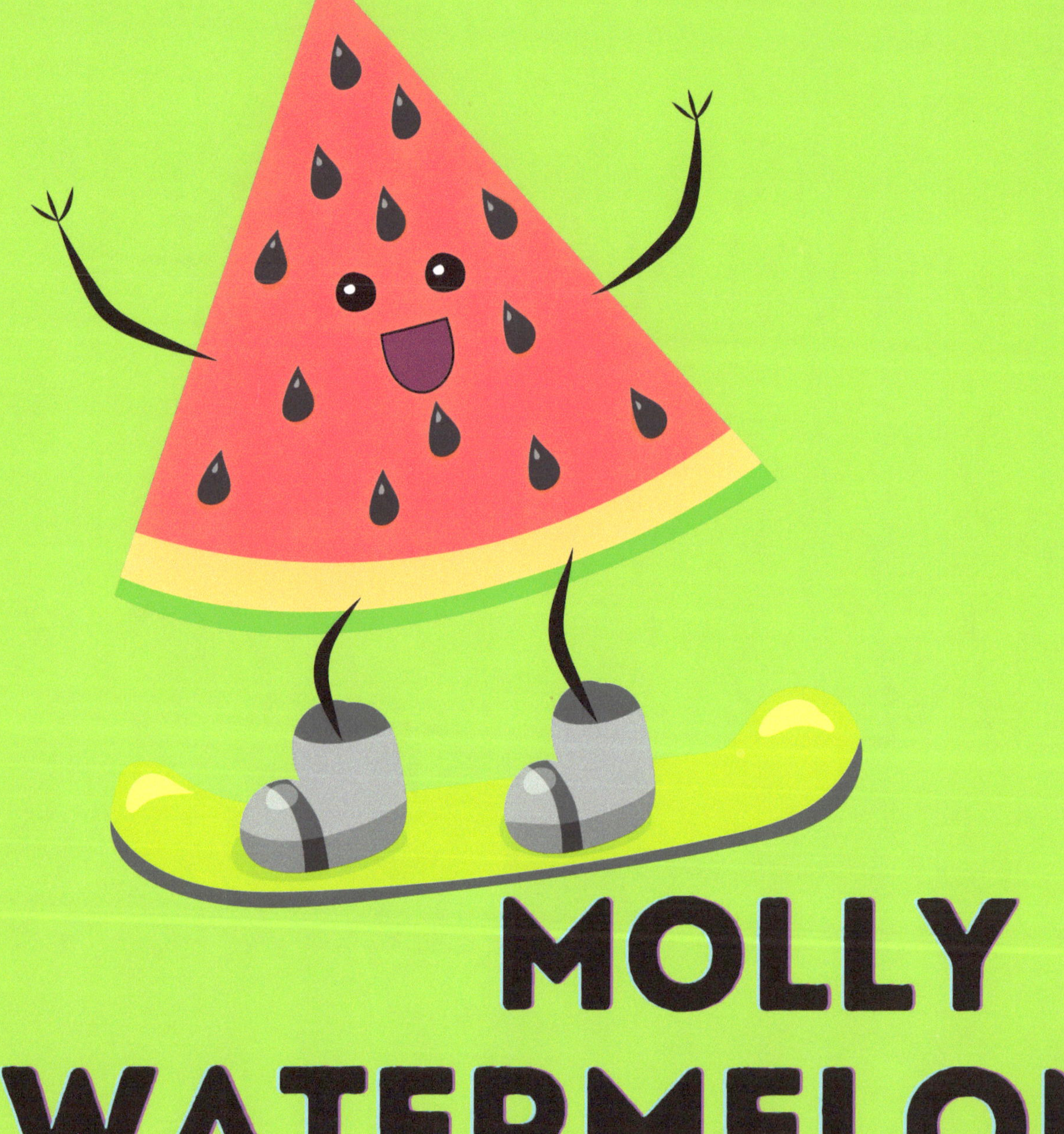

MOLLY
WATERMELON

WATERMELON IS GOOD FOR YOUR SKIN AND EYES.

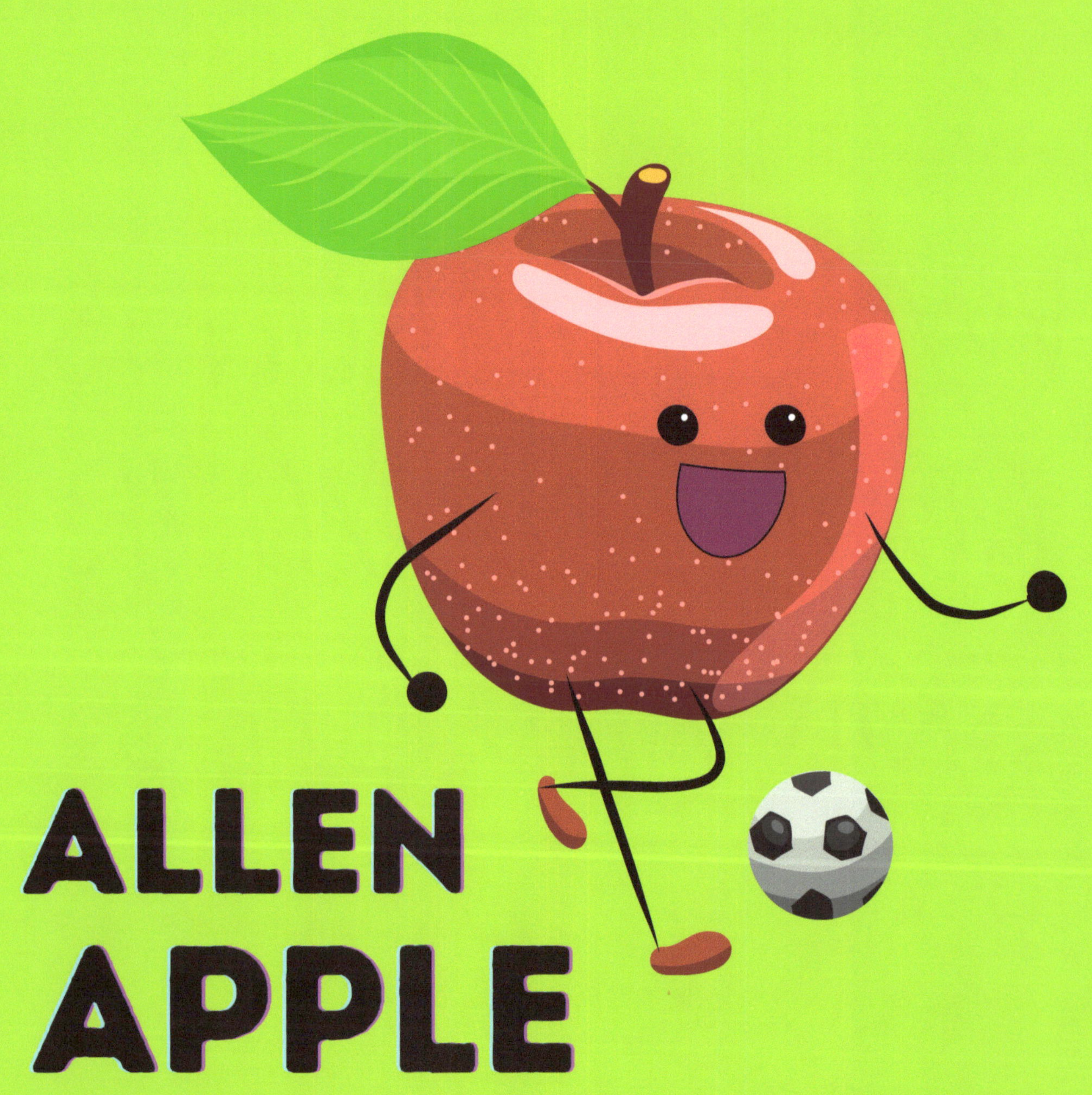

ALLEN
APPLE

APPLES ARE
GOOD FOR YOUR
TEETH AND
HEART.

PATTY PEAR

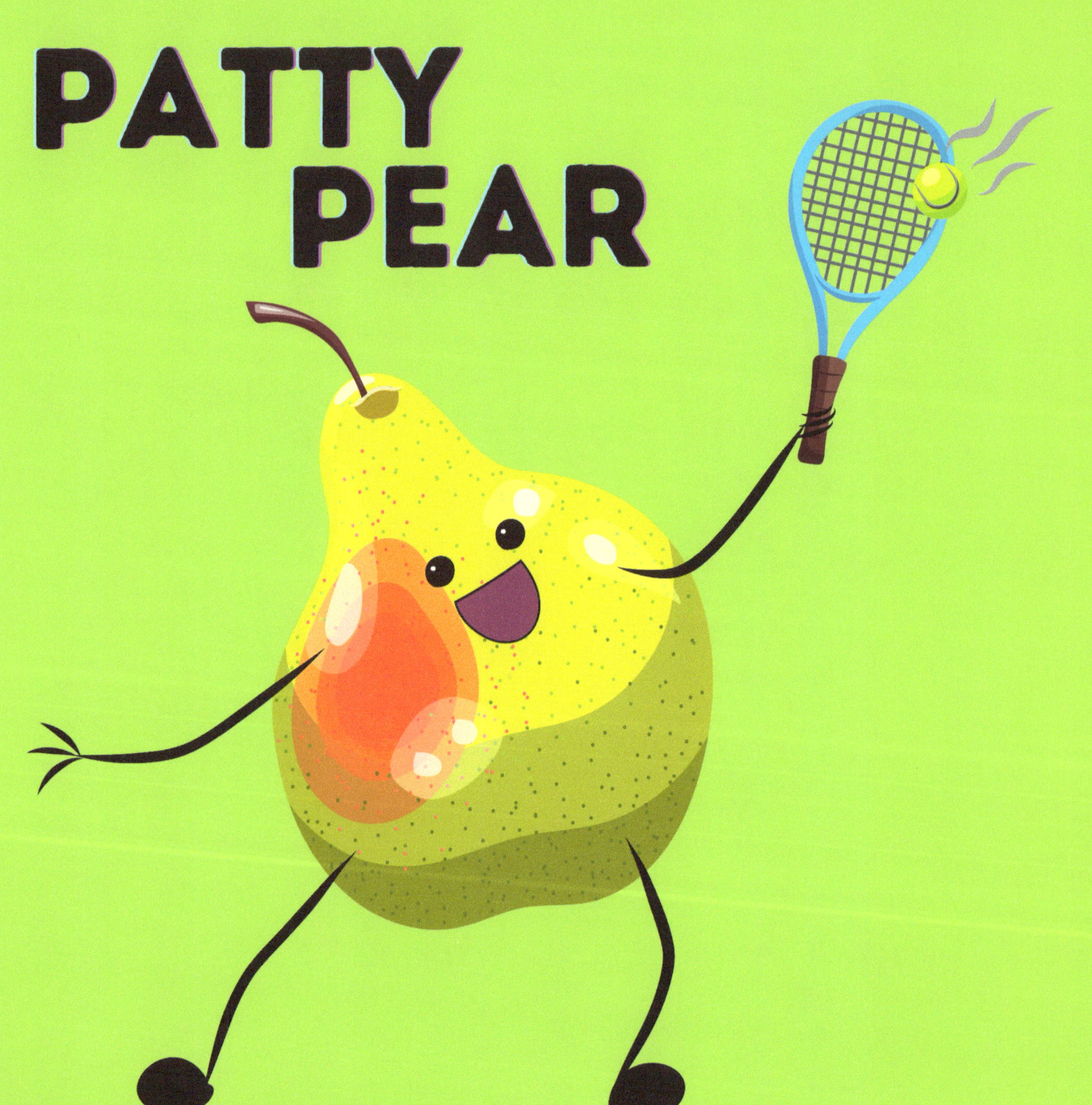

PEARS HELP
WITH POTTY TIME
AND ARE GOOD
FOR YOUR HEART.

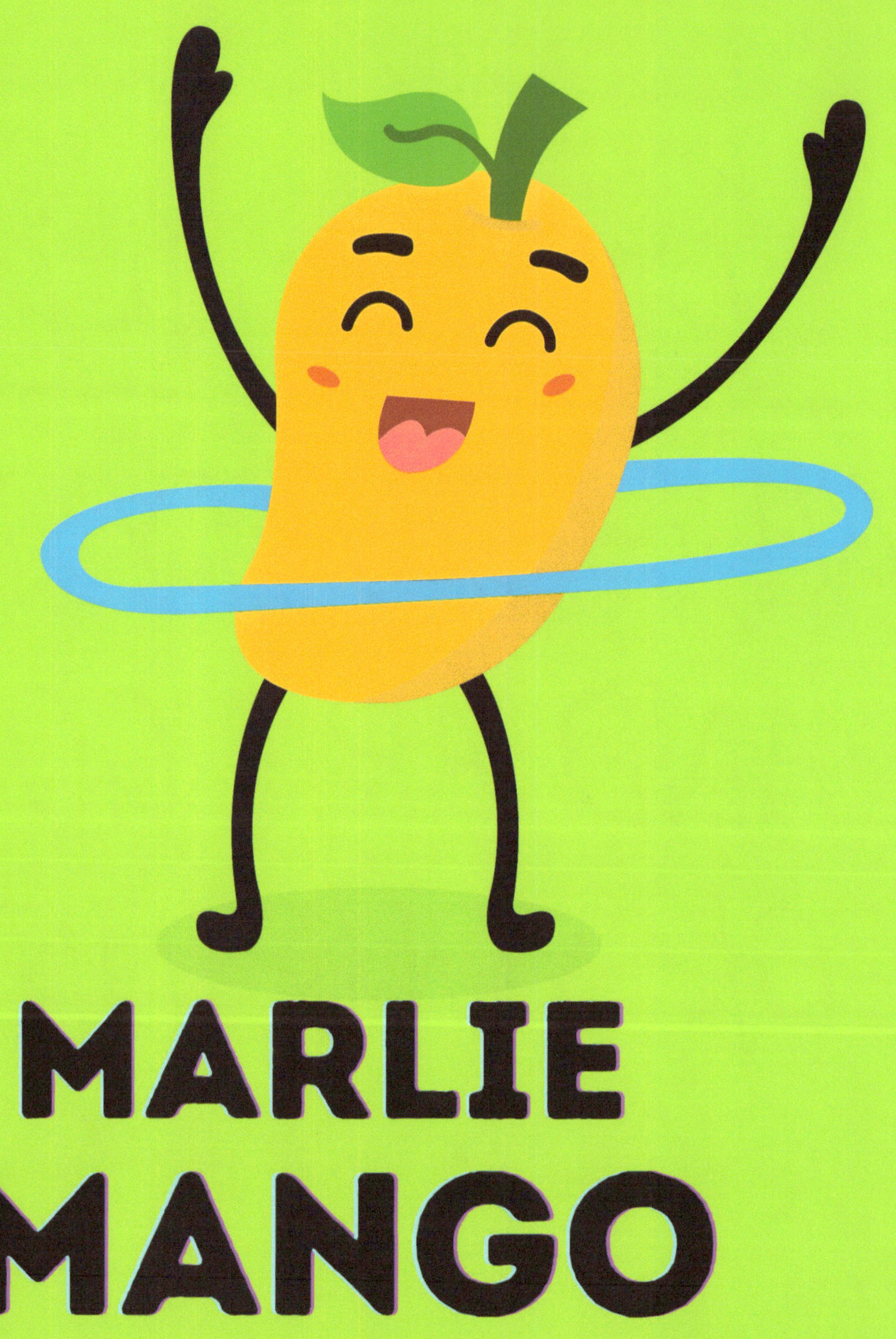

MARLIE
MANGO

MANGOES ARE GOOD FOR THE HEART AND EYES.

KYLA KIWI

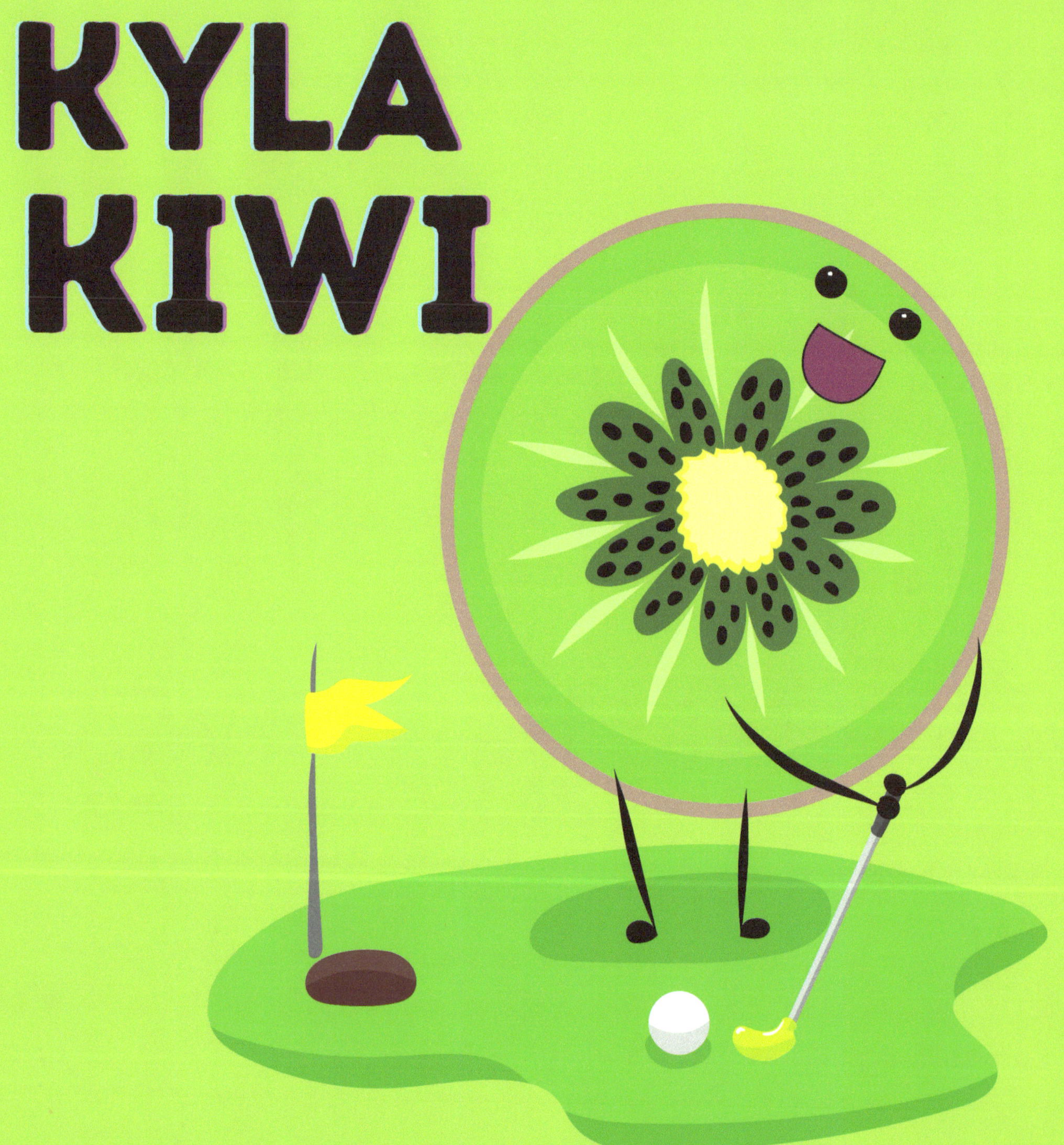

KIWI IS GOOD FOR
NAP TIME AND
YOUR EYES.

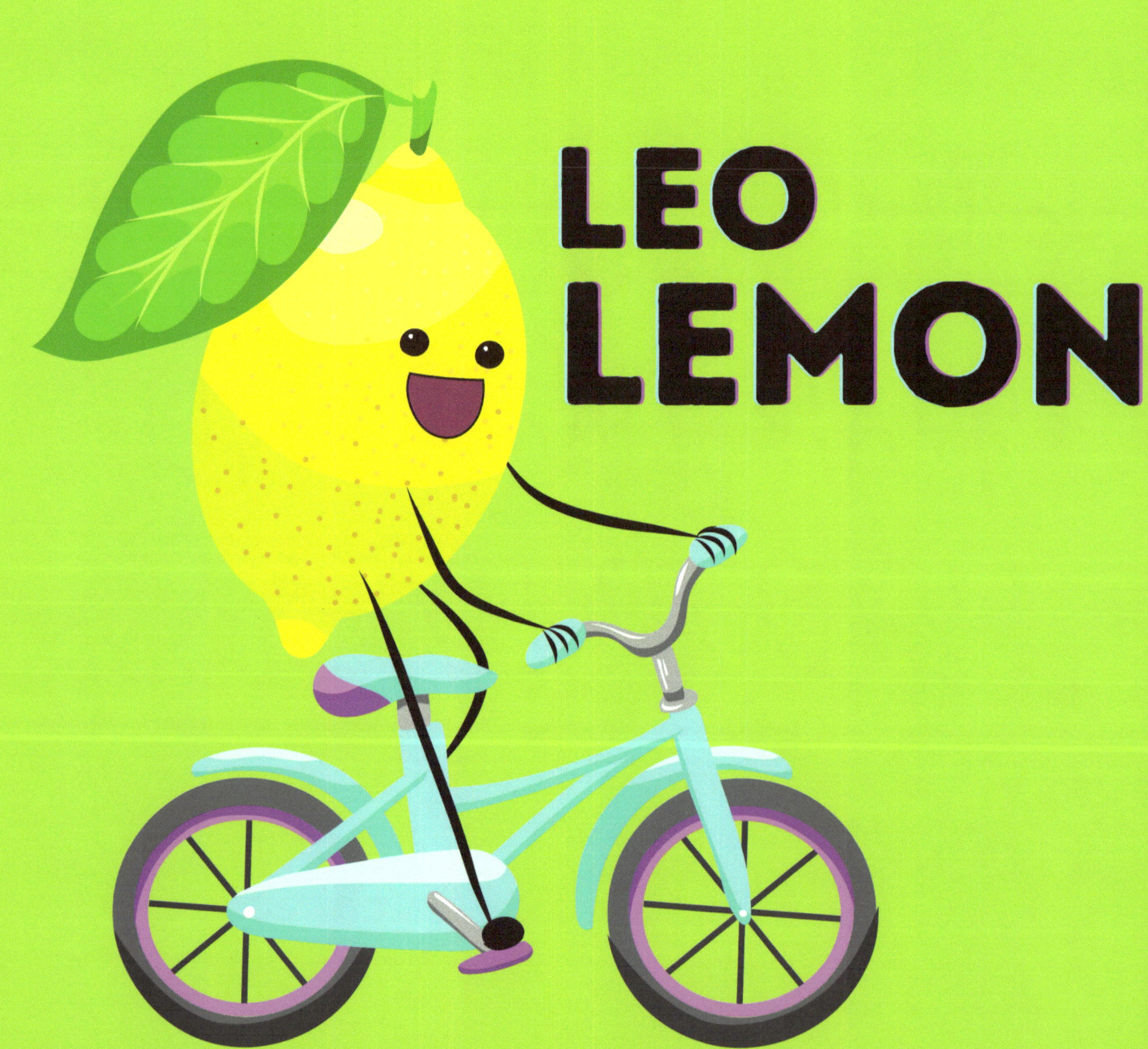
LEO
LEMON

LEMONS HELP WITH DIGESTION AND POTTY TIME.

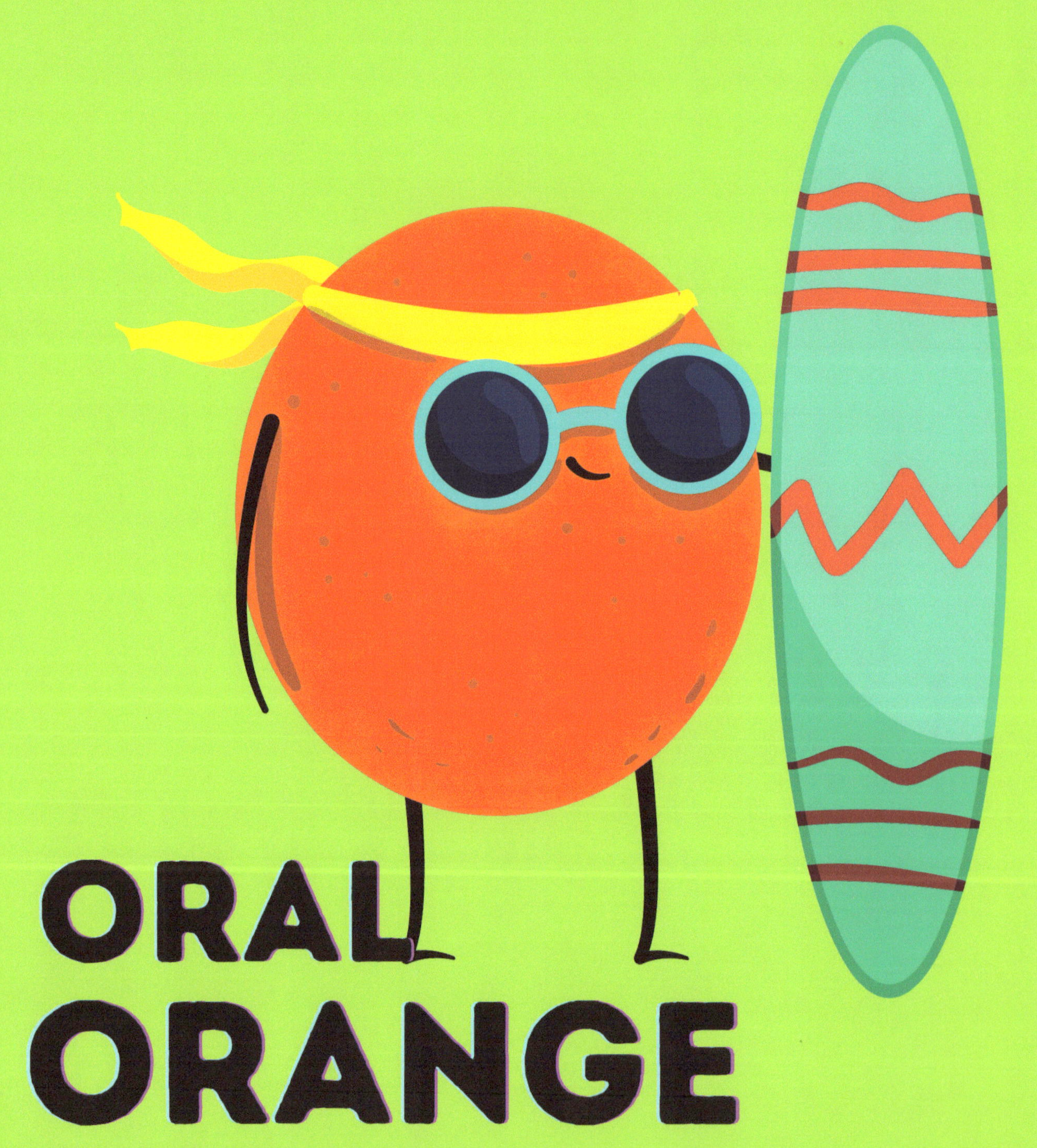

ORAL
ORANGE

ORANGES ARE GOOD FOR YOUR SKIN AND HELP TO PREVENT COLDS.

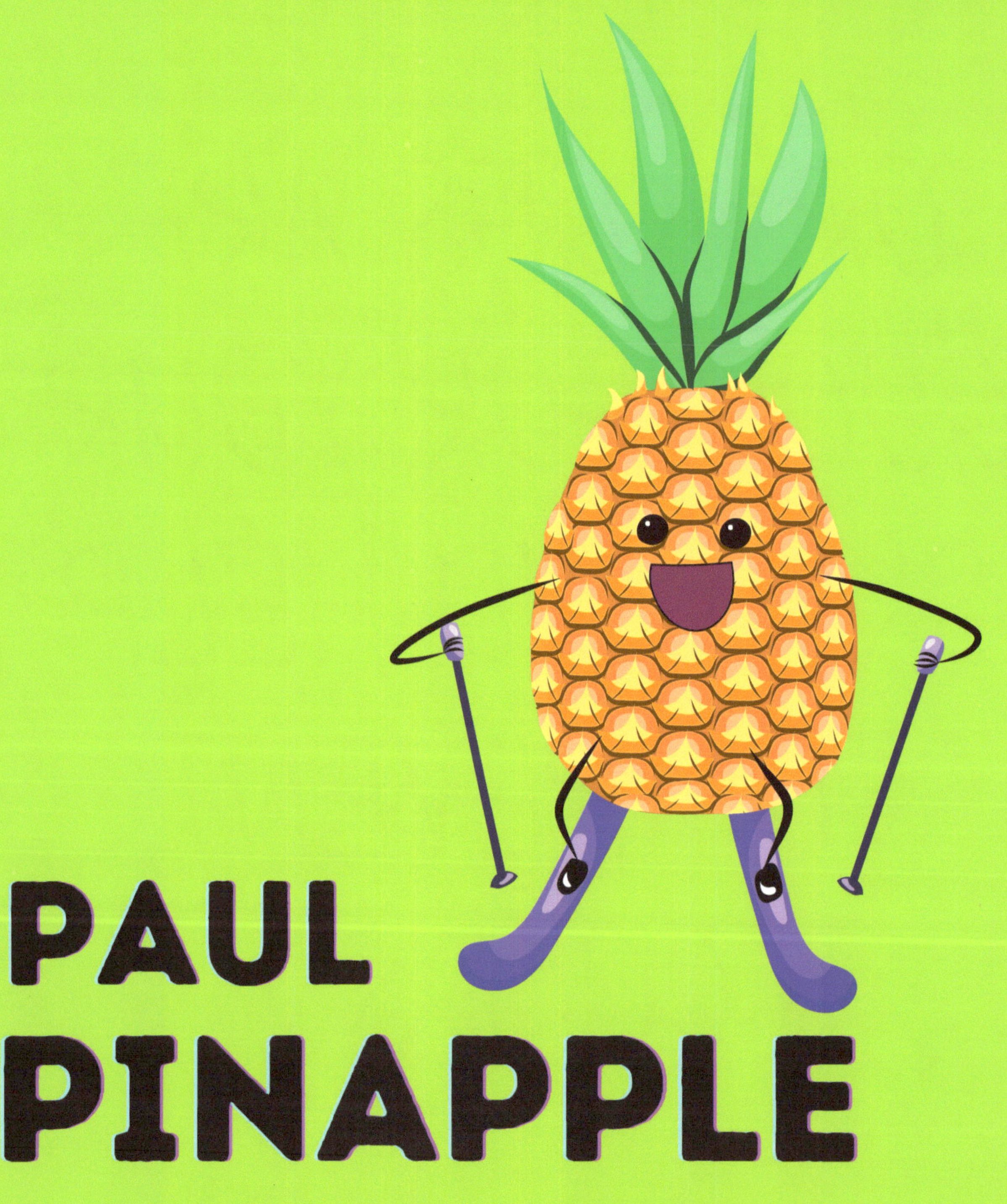

PAUL PINAPPLE

PINEAPPLES HELP WITH DIGESTION AND SIGNS OF COUGHS AND COLDS.

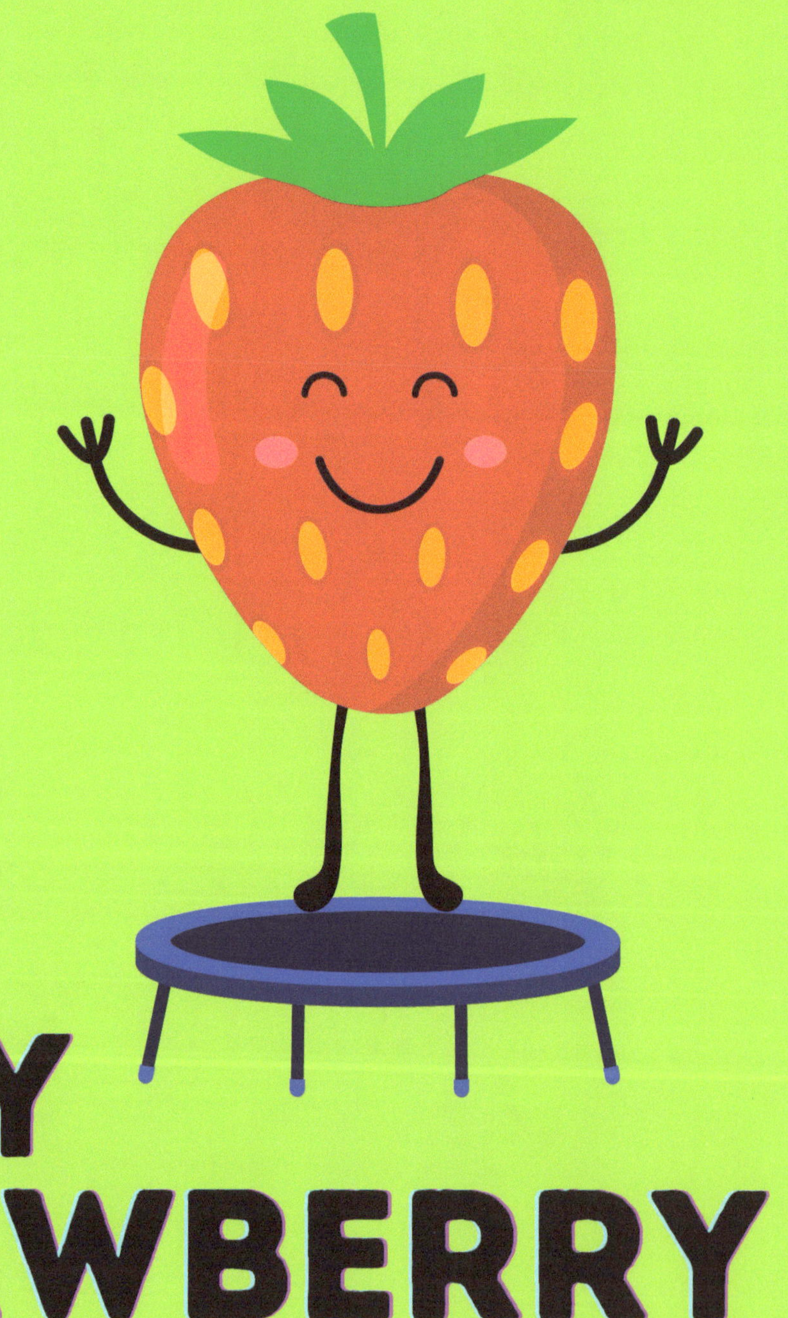

SALLY STRAWBERRY

STRAWBERRIES ARE GOOD FOR THE HEART AND SKIN.

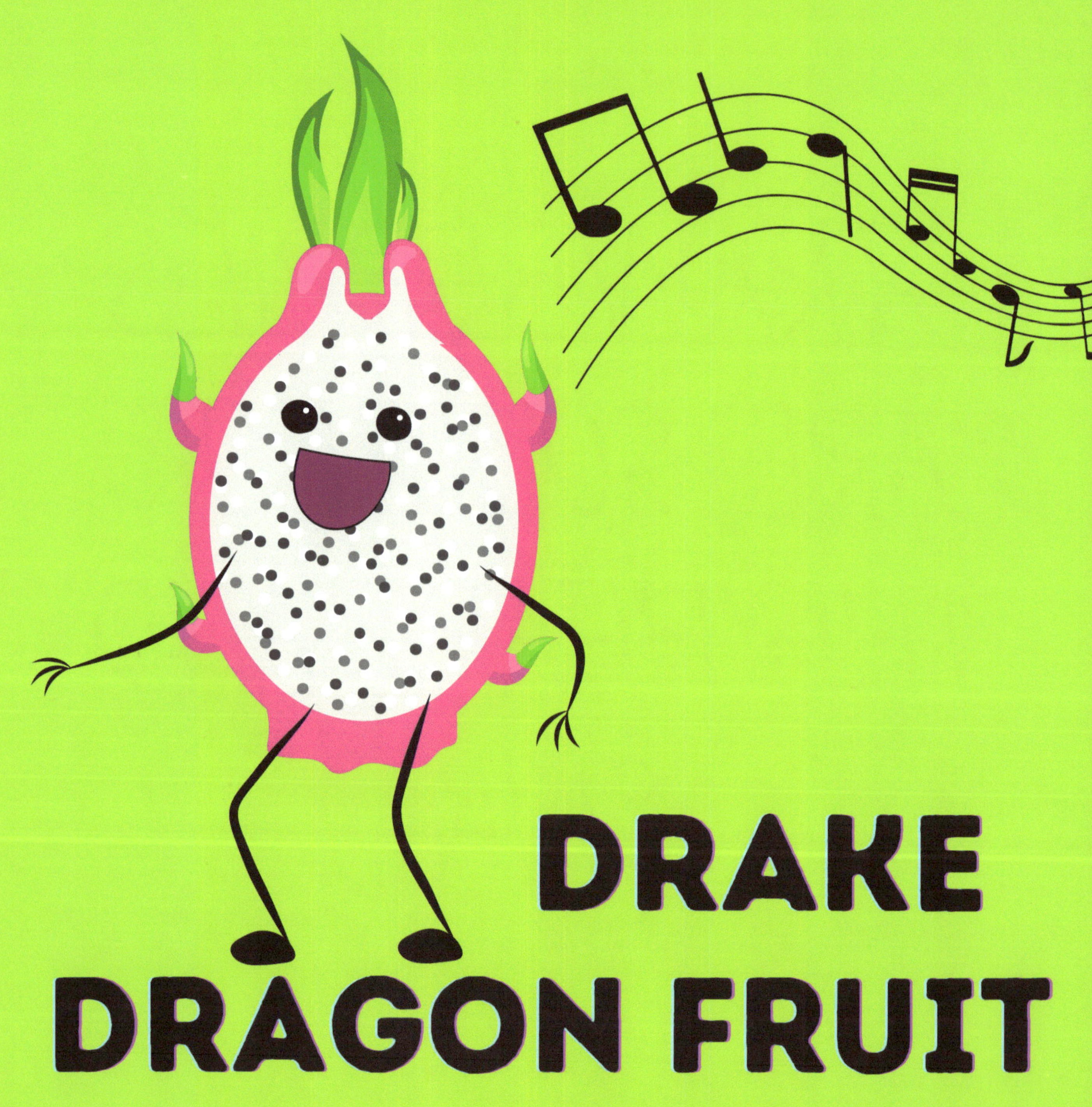

DRAKE
DRAGON FRUIT

DRAGON FRUIT
GIVES YOU
ENERGY AND IS
GOOD FOR THE
BRAIN.

NOW LET'S GO SHOPPING.

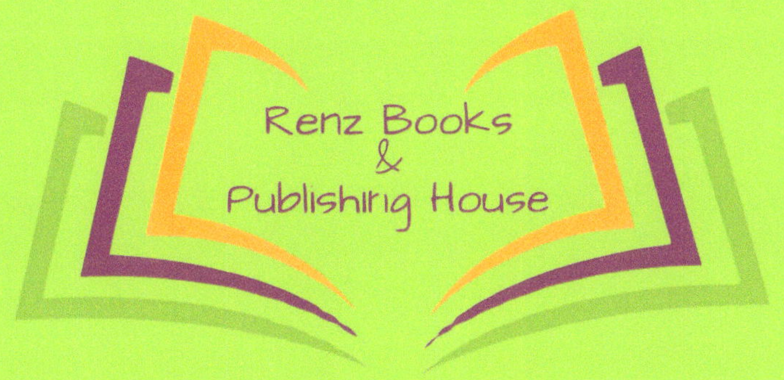
Renz Books
&
Publishing House